Dedication:

I would like to take this time and thank the Good Lord for giving us this opportunity to create such a wonderful diabetic cookbook. I could not have done it without all of the great recipes from the following people:

Recipes written and donated by:

Jim Taylor
Linda Scruggs
Christina Roberts
Anonymous Givers

Articles written by:

Georgina Jones

Thank you all and God Bless!!

ISBN: 978-1-257-08942-0

Table of Contents:

Diabetes

What is this thing they call Diabetes? Why does it control our bodies? What does it have to do with what we eat?

Well, we all know that living with diabetes is no fun, but as long as you understand what it is and give it the respect it demands, the better off you will begin to feel.

Diabetes is a disease. It's a disease that makes the body unable to use its insulin properly. When this happens the glucose remains in your bloodstream instead of being absorbed by cells and used for energy, then the glucose levels in your blood can rise dangerously high. Overtime it can cause damage to your major organs such as; the kidneys, the eyes, the nerves, and the blood vessels, unless you seek help. Getting some advice from your family physician will ease your mind and help you manage your diabetes without stressing out.

There are three forms of diabetes that you can get. There is Type I (also known as Juvenile Diabetes), Type II, and Gestational Diabetes. Below is a short description of each to help you better understand each one.

Type I diabetes is the most serious but least common form. It is also known as Juvenile diabetes, because it mainly affects children and adolescents. People with Type 1 diabetes cannot make enough hormone insulin in their pancreas that they need to help glucose (energy) get into the body's cells. They will need to take insulin and to balance their food intake with insulin.

Now **Type II diabetes** is the most common and usually develops after age 40. Type II diabetes is more likely to develop if you are overweight and have high blood pressure, high levels of fat in your blood, or a history of diabetes in your family. The treatment is weight loss and increased physical activity, sometimes along with medication (pills or insulin injections). Type II is even rising rapidly in children. Parents, we need to get outside with our children and play. It's free to throw the ball in the back yard and everyone has fun in the process.

And last but not least there is the **Gestational diabetes.** This kind of diabetes develops in some women during pregnancy. Which is why all pregnant women should be tested for diabetes between 24 and 28 weeks of pregnancy so that gestational diabetes, if found, can be treated.

 Women who are overweight and older are more likely to have gestational diabetes, too.

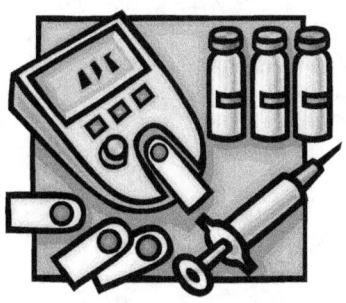

CLASSIC SYMPTOMS OF DIABETES

Learning to recognize the symptoms of diabetes is an important way to detect the condition early. Often times there are no symptoms at all and your diabetes is simply diagnosed by a routine blood or urine test. When these symptoms finally present themselves, they will usually have a classic appearance, such as; excessive urination, frequent trips to the bathroom in the middle of the night, intense thirst, hunger, and severe fatigue. Other symptoms may include: dry skin, blurred vision, unexplained weight loss and a malnourished appearance.

There are certain symptoms that can indicate when your blood glucose reading is not regulated. For example when levels are too high, you might experience: frequent urination, increased thirst, fatigue, and pain in the abdomen.

Certain events can also cause your blood glucose levels to drop low. If your glucose levels are too low, you might experience: shakiness, dizziness, sweating, hunger, headache, pale skin color, behavior changes, jerky movements, seizures, difficulty paying attention, confusion, and or tingling sensations around the mouth. To make matters even more confusing, your blood glucose level may be affected by factors such as; illness, exercising, stress, and excessive heat.

But not all people are the same; some people with diabetes might not experience any symptoms, while others might have very different symptoms than any of those listed above. Remember these symptoms listed are not a diagnostic for diabetes, so if you have any of the symptoms listed you should contact your doctor to schedule an appointment to have a test done. Better safe than sorry!

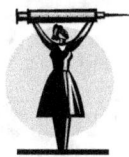

Questions for the doctor

Okay you've gone to the doctor and he has diagnosed you with diabetes. What Now?

Well, the obvious first questions would be:

1. What is diabetes?
2. How did I get it?

But by now all questions have gone blank and you feel stunned by the news. The doctor sends you home. What should you do now?
You could sit back and worry about the problem or you can stand up and take control of your diabetes. To take control, you'll need to write down a list of questions you want answered about diabetes and go back to see your doctor.

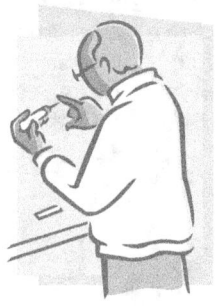

Here is a complied list of questions to help you get some answers from your doctor.

Begin with asking:

How can I improve my blood sugar control?

How often and under what conditions should I test my blood sugar?

What is my hemoglobin?

What is a normal hemoglobin?

How can I get my hemoglobin in the normal range?

What should I do with the results? When should I get together with a dietitian to review what I eat?

What exercises are best for me?

What adjustments to my food or insulin should I make if I plan to exercise?

What effect has diabetes had on my eyes and kidneys?

How should I take care of my feet?

What should my family and friends do if my blood sugar goes so low that I need their help?

Are there any diabetes groups that I could attend in our area?

(For women)

What should I do about taking care of my diabetes if I plan to become or are pregnant?

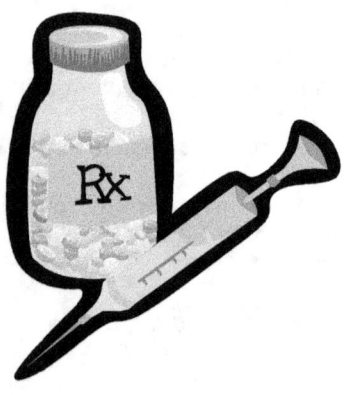

Meal Planning

The first thing people think of when you mention diabetes is that you will have to give up everything with sugar in it for the rest of your life.

Okay, stop right there, that is not true, but what you do need to do as soon as you are diagnosed is to meet with a dietitian or diabetes educator who specializes in meal planning. Every person's meal plan will be different depending on their backgrounds, and other medical conditions that they may have. So, if you need to lose weight or to gain weight than this will be the person who will know how to do it correctly. A dietitian will also teach you how to maintain your weight and how to count carbohydrate grams or to use the diabetic exchange and finally how to become a savvy food shopper and read labels for not only your health, but for your family as well.

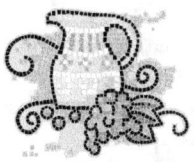

Your meal plan that you and your dietitian should design, will include:

- The number of meals you consume per day
- Portions of meals (whether 3 big meals or numerous small meals)
- The number of calories that you will need to eat
- The number of calories that you have consumed
- What special foods you can have and on which days
- How to correctly add sugar to your recipes
- Guidelines on how to lower fat and cholesterol intake
- Guidelines on how to dine out and drink a glass of wine with your meals

One more thing you need to learn form your dietitian is how to read the labels of food before you just eat it. A savvy shopper can learn to feed the whole family with delicious dinners instead of a bland boring meal.

What to eat?

Since the beginning, we have discussed what diabetes is, what the symptoms are, and meal planning. The big question that lies on everyone's tongues is:

Well, what can I eat?

Actually you can eat quite a bit, although there are some foods that you will need to eat in moderation. Remember to get with your dietitian or doctor before changing your diets or medications.

The following list is just a guideline.

Eat 6 servings a day or more of starches such as: bread, cereal, and starchy vegetables.

Dry cereal with non-fat/skim milk
Bagel with one Tsp. of jam
Pasta with tomato sauce
Baked potato with bbq or chili
Try adding cooked black beans, corn, or chickpeas to salads or casseroles.

Eat 5 or more a day of fruits and vegetables.

Grab a piece of fruit for a snack, instead of candy or chips.
Pack raw vegetables for lunch such as: broccoli, carrots, cauliflower, or green bell peppers.
You can also add fresh vegetables to chili, stir-fried dishes, and stews.

Make sure to eat your sugars and sweets in moderation.

Pick your favorite sweets and include them in your meal plan as a special food treat, but only do this once or twice a week at the very most.
Split a dessert with your friend to satisfy your sweet tooth. This will also lower the sugar, fat, and calories you will be consuming.

Learn to eat less total fat by using:

Low-fat or fat-free cream cheese, salad dressing, mayonnaise, or sour cream.
Also try using less:

butter/margarine, salad dressing, or oil.

Never "Sauté" with butter, instead try "Sautéing" with flavored vinegars or lemon/lime juice and when cooking with oil, choose olive, canola, soybean, corn, sunflower, and or safflower oils.

Eat less saturated fat.

Choose lean cuts of meats, such as: beef, lamb, pork, or veal.

Treat the meat as the side dish and not the main course, by chopping up into a salad or casserole.

Eat more skinless poultry and seafood prepared by grilling or broiling. (Never eat the skin of a chicken. It is totally saturated fat.) Try using low-fat dairy products. Non-fat/skim milk, low-fat cheeses, low-fat yogurt, and low-fat dairy desserts is a great way to start. Moderate your intake of foods for several days by keeping a food diary. This will help you see your progress, so you can begin to feel better.

Breads

Stuffed French toast

1 loaf French bread
½ lb. ham, sliced thin
1 pkg. Light American cheese
½ c. Skim milk
4 egg substitute
1 Tsp. cinnamon
½ lb. Sausage
½ pkg. Bacon
1 ½ Tsp. Vanilla

In large skillet, fry the bacon and sausage together until done. While the meat is cooking, slice the French bread into eight slices and then slice each one ¾ of the way through. Mix the milk, egg sub., cinnamon and vanilla together into a batter in a deep bowl and set it to the side. Place the cooked bacon and sausage on a paper towel and drain. Divide into eight equal parts and do the same with the ham. Dip each piece of bread into the batter and submerge it so that both sides are coated. Open each piece and put in one portion of bacon, sausage, ham and cheese, then close the bread. Fry the stuffed batter coated bread slices in the skillet. Cook until golden brown on the outside and making sure the cheese is melted on the inside.

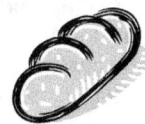

Herb Bread

1 ½ c. whole wheat flour
1 c. of hot water
1 pkg. quick-rise dry yeast
2 Tbls. Canola oil
¼ c. egg substitute at room temperature
¼ c. non-fat dry milk
2 Tbls. sugar
1 ½ c. all-purpose flour
½ Tsp. ground nutmeg
1 Tsp. dried Sage
1 Tbls. low-fat margarine
1 Tsp. Celery Seed
Non-stick Cooking Spray

Combine in a large bowl whole wheat flour, yeast, milk, sugar, nutmeg, sage, and celery seed. Pour in hot water and add oil and egg substitute. Mix thoroughly. Gradually add all-purpose flour, ¼c. at a time, to make moderately soft dough. On a lightly floured surface knead until smooth, about 9 minutes. Place dough in bowl coated with cooking spray and turn to coat. Cover and allow to rise until doubled in bulk, 30 to 45 minutes. Punch down dough and turn onto floured surface. Knead 30 seconds to press out bubbles that have formed throughout dough. Shape dough into round or rectangular loaf and place in pan that has been coated with non-stick cooking spray. Cover with light cloth and allow dough to rise until almost doubled, about 30 minutes. Preheat oven to 375 degrees and bake loaf 30 to 35 minutes or until done. Brush hot loaf with melted margarine.

Seasoned Bread Crumbs

2 c. fine dry bread crumbs
½ c. finely chopped onion
½ c. finely chopped fresh parsley
1 clove garlic, finely chopped
1 tsp oregano

Combine bread crumbs, onion, parsley, garlic, and oregano; mix thoroughly; store in a tightly covered container in the freezer for up to 6 months.

Apple Pancakes

3 eggs
3 Tbls. low-fat Sour Cream
1 apple, finely chopped
3 Tbls. flour
1 Tsp. baking powder
½ Tsp. Cinnamon

Mix the eggs, sour cream, apples, flour, baking powder, and cinnamon in a medium size bowl. Fold mixture until firmly mixed. Cook on hot lightly greased griddle until golden brown.

Spoon Bread with Canadian bacon

Low-fat butter-flavored cooking spray
2 ounces Canadian bacon, chopped
1/3 c. yellow cornmeal
2/3 c. water
1 Tbls. low-fat margarine
¼ c. egg substitute
1/3 c. skim milk

Preheat the oven to 425°F. Coat a baking dish with cooking spray. Lightly coat a non-stick skillet with cooking spray. Add the bacon and sauté over high heat for 2 minutes. Set aside. Place the cornmeal and water in a small non-stick pot. Bring to a boil. Stir and cook for 1 minute, then remove from the heat. Stir in the margarine, egg substitute, and milk; in that order. Add the reserved Canadian bacon. Spoon the mixture into the prepared baking dish. Bake for about 15 minutes, until set and browned around the edges. Serve warm.

Pumpkin Bread

1 can pumpkin
1 c. sugar
¼ c. vegetable oil
1 c. plain low-fat yogurt
1 ½ c. all purpose flour
1 ½ c. whole wheat flour
2 Tsp. baking powder
2 Tsp. baking soda
2 Tsp. cinnamon
½ Tsp. salt
1 c. raisins

Preheat oven to 350 degrees. In a large mixing bowl, beat together pumpkin, sugar, oil, and yogurt. In a medium bowl, combine the flours, baking powder, soda, cinnamon, and salt; add to pumpkin mixture, stirring until just moistened. Stir in raisins. Pour into 2 greased 9x5x3 inch loaf pans and bake for about 1 hour. Cool on a wire rack for 10 minutes; remove from pan and cool completely.

Navajo Fry Bread

2 c. flour
4 Tsp. baking powder
1 Tsp. Salt
2/3 c. warm water
Oil

Put 2 to 3 inches of oil in frying pan and heat to 400 degrees. Combine the flour, baking powder, and salt in bowl. Add ½c. of warm water and continue adding water to reach the consistency of bread dough. Tear off into balls of dough. Roll out balls on a board lightly dusted with cornmeal to ¼ inch thick. Punch a hole in the center of each piece. Fry bread one at a time, turning as soon as it becomes golden. Drain on paper towel and serve hot.

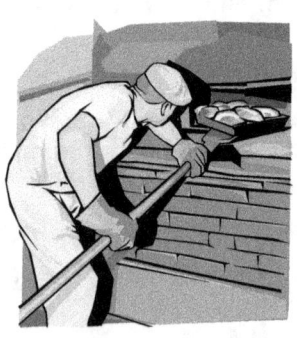

Appetizers

Snacks: A Healthy Necessity in a Diabetic Diet

Snacks play a very important role in the daily life of a person with diabetes, particularly those with Type 1 diabetes and insulin-requiring Type 2 diabetes. For these people between meal and bedtime snacks are essential to keep blood glucose levels as close to normal as possible and to help prevent low blood sugar (hypoglycemia).
Wherever you go you should always carry a supply of snacks to eat in case of low blood sugar. Make sure to keep snacks in your purse, the glove compartment of your car, or in your office desk drawer.

Here's a list of snacks that can be
purchased at most supermarkets.

Apples
Fresh apricots
Bananas
Cantaloupe
Cherries
Dried dates
Dried figs
Gingersnaps
Graham crackers
Low-fat Granola bars
Grapes
Kumquats
Nectarines
Skim milk
Oranges
Peaches
Peanut butter sandwich crackers
Pear
Plums
Popcorn, low-fat
Prunes
Pretzels
Raisins
Rice cakes
Saltine crackers
Tangerines
Vanilla Wafers
Non-fat yogurt, plain or fruit

Taco Popcorn

7 ½ c. air-popped popcorn
butter-flavored cooking spray
1 ½ Tsp. cumin
1 ½ Tsp. garlic powder
1 ½ Tsp. onion powder
1 ½ Tsp. Worcestershire sauce
cayenne pepper (optional)

Preheat oven to 300 degrees. Put popcorn in a large mixing bowl and lightly coat popcorn with cooking spray. Toss and coat again. Combine cumin, garlic powder, onion powder, and cayenne pepper. Sprinkle spices over popcorn and toss to coat evenly. Drizzle Worcestershire sauce over popcorn and toss again. Spread popcorn evenly in large baking pan. Bake for 10 minutes, tossing once.
Divide leftovers into individual serving sizes and put into airtight bags. Next time you're hungry for a snack, you can easily incorporate it into your meal plan.

Seasoned Popcorn:
You can make these treats by
using 3c. of unseasoned popped
corn:

Mexican Popcorn

Put the popcorn in a large bowl and
lightly coat with refrigerated
butter-flavored cooking spray.

Combine:

1 Tbls. dried Mexican spiced salad
dressing mix
¼ Tsp. crushed dried oregano
¼ Tsp. crushed dried thyme
¼ Tsp. garlic powder

Sprinkle over popcorn and lightly
coat with additional cooking spray.
Toss again and serve.

Spicy and Sweet Popcorn

Preheat oven to 300°F
Spread popcorn on a non-stick
cookie sheet and lightly coat with
refrigerated butter-flavored
cooking spray.

Combine:

2 ½ Tbls. spoon-able sugar
substitute
¼ Tsp. ground cinnamon
1/8 Tsp. ground nutmeg
¼ Tsp. dried orange peel.

Sprinkle over the popcorn and
toss. Lightly coat again with
cooking spray and toss. Bake for
10 minutes, tossing once. Serve
warm.

Italian Popcorn

Preheat oven to 300 degrees.
Spread popcorn on a non-stick
cookie sheet and lightly coat with
refrigerated butter-flavored
cooking spray.

Mix together:

1 Tsp. crushed dried Italian herbs
1/8 Tsp. cayenne pepper
1 Tsp. grated Parmesan cheese.

Sprinkle over popcorn and lightly
coat again with cooking spray. Toss
and bake for 10 minutes. Serve
warm.

Asian Popcorn

Preheat oven to 250 degrees. Spread popcorn on a non-stick cookie sheet and lightly coat with refrigerated butter-flavored cooking spray.

Mix together:

1 Tbls. low-sodium soy sauce
2 Tsp. fresh lemon juice
1 Tsp. five-spice powder
¼ Tsp. ground coriander
¼ Tsp. garlic powder

Drizzle over popcorn. Toss to coat evenly. Bake 10 minutes. Serve warm.

Orange Popcorn

Put the popcorn in a large bowl and lightly coat with refrigerated butter-flavored cooking spray.

Combine:

2 ½ Tbls. orange-flavored powdered drink mix (already sweetened with sugar substitute) ½ Tsp. dried orange peel.

Toss and coat again with cooking spray.

Apple Dip

8 oz. low-fat Cream Cheese, softened
½ c. fat –free Yogurt
2 medium size Apples, chopped
½ c. chopped Walnuts
1 Tbls. Lemon Juice

Blend together cheese and yogurt. Add the apples, nuts, and lemon juice. Serve with unsalted crackers or bread.

Tomato Basil Pizza Snack

½ whole wheat English muffin
2 Tbls. no added sodium tomato sauce
2 Tbls. low-fat mozzarella cheeses
1 Tbls. fresh basil, chopped
2 Tsp. tomato, diced

Preheat broiler. Place English muffin on a small baking sheet. Spread tomato sauce over top of muffin. Top with cheese. Sprinkle fresh basil and tomato on top. Broil until cheese is brown and sauce is bubbly. Serve immediately.

Tomato Crescents

½ c. warm water
¼ c. Olive oil
¼ c. red vinegar
1 egg substitute
1 Tsp. salt
3 c. flour
1 lb. Low-fat mozzarella cheese
2 large tomatoes, chopped
¼ c. fresh basil, chopped
Paprika to taste

Blend water, oil, vinegar, egg sub., and salt in large bowl. Gradually stir in enough flour so dough pulls away from sides of bowl. Turn dough out onto lightly floured surface and knead until smooth. Shape dough into round. Grease the bowl and add the dough, turning to coat. Cover with damp towel and let stand in warm area for 30 minutes. Preheat oven to 350 F. Grease baking sheets with non-stick spray. Combine cheese, tomatoes, and basil in bowl. Divide dough into 8 pieces. Shape each into smooth round, rolling each out on floured surface to thickness of ¼ inch. Spoon some of the cheese mixture down center of each round. Fold one side over filling; press edges to seal. Arrange crescents on prepared baking sheets. Sprinkle with paprika and bake until cheese has melted and pastry is golden brown, 40 minutes.

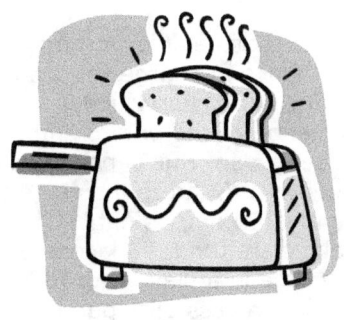

SOUP

Creamy Seven Soup

1 c. of Cauliflower
1 c. of Broccoli
1 small Carrot
1 small White Turnip
¼ small Cabbage
1 medium Potato
½ c. green peas
5 c. chicken broth
1 tbsp chopped fresh parsley

Wash and chop cauliflower and broccoli. Place in a large saucepan. Wash, peel, and chop carrot, turnip, cabbage and potato and add to saucepan. Stir in peas and chicken broth. Bring to a boil, and boil gently 20 minutes until vegetables are tender. Place about 2c. at a time in a blender or food processor; process until pureed and smooth. You can refrigerate it at this time. Serve hot or chilled, garnished with chopped parsley.

Chunky Chicken and Vegetable Soup

1 Tbls. canola oil
1 boneless skinless chicken breast, chopped in bite size pieces
½ c. chopped green bell pepper
½ c. thinly sliced celery
2 green onions, sliced
2 cans chicken broth
1 c. water
½ c. sliced carrots
1 Tbls. finely chopped fresh parsley
¼ Tsp. dried thyme leaves
1/8 Tsp. black pepper

Pre-heat oil in large saucepan; add chicken and cook over medium heat; stirring 4 to 5 minutes or until chicken is no longer pink. Add the bell pepper, celery and onions. Cook and stir 7 minutes or until vegetables are tender. Add broth, water, carrots, parsley, thyme, and black pepper. Simmer 10 minutes or until carrots are tender.

Creamy Peanut Butter Soup
Non-stick cooking spray

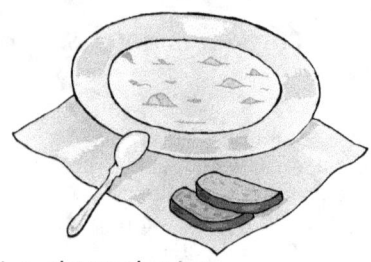

½ c. chopped onion
½ c. chopped carrot
½ c. sliced celery
2 cloves garlic, minced
3 c. reduced-sodium chicken broth
1 can northern beans, drained
½ c. reduced-fat peanut butter
½ c. skim milk
½ tsp curry powder
2 to 3 tsp lemon juice
1 to 2 sprints of hot pepper sauce
Salt, cayenne, and black pepper, to taste
Thinly sliced green onion, as garnish

Spray large saucepan with cooking spray; heat over medium heat until hot, then sauté onion, carrot, celery, and garlic for 5 minutes. Add the chicken broth and beans; heat to boiling. Reduce heat and simmer, covered, until vegetables

are tender, 10 to 15 minutes.
Process soup and peanut butter in
food processor until smooth.
Return soup to saucepan; stir in
the skim milk and curry powder.
Heat over medium heat until hot.
Season to taste with lemon juice,
hot pepper sauce, salt, cayenne,
and black pepper. Pour soup into
bowls; sprinkle with green onion
and low-fat shredded cheese.

Zesty Chili

4 pounds round steak, cut into small
cubes
4 garlic cloves, minced
¼ c. olive oil
3 c. chopped onion
2 ¾ c. water, divided
2 c. sliced celery
3 cans diced tomatoes
2 cans no-salt tomato sauce
1 jar salsa
3 Tbsp chili powder
2 tsp ground cumin
2 tsp dried oregano
1 tsp pepper
¼ c. all-purpose flour
¼ c. yellow cornmeal

In a Dutch oven over medium-high heat, sauté steak and garlic in oil until browned.

Add onion; cook and stir for 5 minutes.

Stir in 2 c. water and next eight ingredients; bring to a boil.

Reduce the heat; cover and simmer for 2 hours or until tender.

Combine flour, cornmeal and remaining water; stir until smooth. Bring chili to a boil.

Add flour mixture; cook and stir 2 minutes or until thickened.

If desired, garnish with low-fat cheese, light sour cream, onions and or olives.

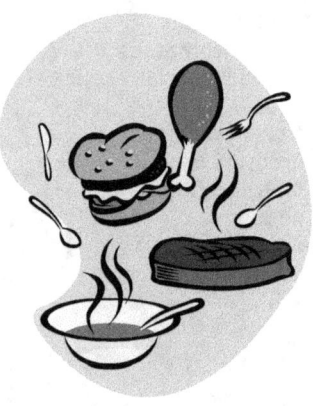

Sandwiches

Sloppy Joes

1 lb. extra-lean ground beef
¼ c. tomato juice
2 Tbls. green onions
1 Tbls. prepared mustard
¼ Tsp. dry mustard
2 Tbls. ketchup
½ Tsp. salt

Brown the ground beef in canola oil. Add the onions and sauté. Drain off the remaining fat. Mix the remaining ingredients together and stir into the beef and onions. Simmer for 20 to 30 minutes, stirring occasionally. Serve on a sesame seed bun.

Baked Grilled Cheese Sandwiches

Non-stick cooking spray
2 egg whites
2 Tbls. fat-free milk
4 slices fat-free cheese

2 dash of paprika
Kosher dill pickle
4 slices wheat bread

Preheat oven to 400 degrees. Take a whisk and a shallow bowl and mix; the egg whites, fat-free milk, and paprika together. Dip each side of the bread in the egg mixture and place on a baking sheet that has been coated with non-stick cooking spray. Bake until toasted brown on both sides. When golden brown, top each piece of bread with cheese and allow to melt slightly. Place on serving plates, eat warm, and top with kosher pickle.

Club Wrap

low-fat whole wheat tortilla
2 Tsp. light cream cheese
1 oz. lean turkey slice
1 oz. lean ham slice
low-fat Swiss cheese
green leaf lettuce leaf
3 tomato slices

Place tortilla on a flat surface. Spread cream cheese on one side of the tortilla. Lay the lettuce, turkey, ham, Swiss cheese, and tomato on top of the cream cheese on the flat tortilla. Bring the sides of the wrap in and then roll up in the shape of a cylinder. Wrap each in plastic wrap until ready to serve. Right before serving, slice wraps in half, and remove plastic wrap.

Chunky Chicken Sandwiches

non-stick cooking spray
1 small onion sliced thin
4 ounces mushrooms, sliced thin
1 clove garlic, minced
1 Tbls. low fat Ranch Dressing
2 Tsp. ketchup
¼ Tsp. Dijon mustard
4 boneless, chicken breasts
4 wheat rolls cut in half

Preheat grill or broiler. Coat your skillet with non-stick cooking spray. Sauté the onions and mushrooms over medium high heat until they are cooked through and begin to brown. Add the garlic and roast for two more minutes. Set to the side. In a small bowl combine the dressing, ketchup, and mustard. Set to the side. Grill the chicken until done. Allow to stand for 5 minutes then cut into thin slices. Place 1 Tsp. of the sauce on the bottom of each roll. Top with chicken slices, onions and mushrooms. Serve warm.

Southwestern Sloppy Joes

1 pound lean ground beef round
1 c. chopped onion
¼ c. chopped celery
¼ c. water
1 can diced tomatoes and green chilies, un-drained
1 can no-salt tomato sauce
½ Tsp. ground cumin
¼ Tsp. salt
9 wheat hamburger buns

Heat large non-stick skillet over high heat; add beef, onion, celery, and water. Reduce heat to medium. Cook and stir 5 minutes or until meat is no longer pink. Drain fat and rinse with water. Stir in tomatoes and green chilies, tomato sauce, cumin, and salt; bring to a boil over high heat. Reduce heat; simmer 20 minutes or until mixture thickens. Serve on wheat buns.

Tuna Salad Melt Down

1 can chunk tuna packed in water,
drained
¾ c. chopped cabbages
1 small Carrot, shredded
3 Tbls. sliced green onions
3 Tbls. reduced-fat mayonnaise
1 Tbls. Dijon mustard
1 Tsp. dried dill weed
4 wheat rolls or buns, lightly toasted
1/3 c. shredded reduced-fat Cheddar
cheese

Preheat broiler. Combine tuna,
cabbage, carrot, and green onions
in medium bowl. Combine
mayonnaise, mustard, and dill
weed in small bowl. Stir
mayonnaise mixture into tuna
mixture. Spread tuna mixture onto
bun halves. Place on broiler pan
and broil for 3 to 4 minutes or until
heated through. Sprinkle with low-
fat cheese. Broil 1 to 2 minutes
more or until cheese melts.

Jamaican Jerk

1 Tsp. Jerk seasoning (recipe follows)

4 boneless skinless chicken breasts
2 Tbls. reduced-fat mayonnaise
2 Tbls. plain non-fat yogurt
1 Tbls. mango chutney
4 onion rolls, split
4 lettuce leaves
8 slices tomato

Jerk Seasoning:

1 ½ Tsp. salt
1 ½ Tsp. ground allspice
1 Tsp. sugar substitute
1 Tsp. ground dried thyme leaves
1 Tsp. black pepper
½ Tsp. garlic powder
½ Tsp. ground red pepper
¼ Tsp. ground cinnamon
¼ Tsp. ground nutmeg

Combine all ingredients in small bowl.

Prepare Jerk Seasoning.

Roll chicken in the jerk seasoning and coat them evenly. Set on plate and set aside. Spray grill with non-stick cooking spray and prepare it for high cooking. Place chicken on grill, 3 to 4 inches from medium-hot coals. Grill 5 to 7 minutes on each side or until no longer pink in center. Combine the mayonnaise, yogurt, and chutney in small bowl; spread 1 Tablespoonful onto each onion roll. Place chicken on onion roll bottoms; top each with lettuce leaf, 2 slices of tomatoes, and top with roll.

Egg Salad

3 hard boiled eggs
3 oz. low-fat cottage cheese
1 Tsp. mustard
1 tbsp. chopped onion
1 tbsp. dill cubes or pickle relish
salt and pepper to taste
1 freely chopped celery

Boil eggs and set a side to cool. Mix cheese, mustard, onion, relish, and celery together in bowl. Finely chop eggs and add to mixture; stirring well and adding salt and pepper for seasoning to your taste. Makes lunch for two. Good on sandwich with tomato.

Sausage Sandwiches

¼ lb. bulk Italian Sausage
1 Tbls. chopped onion
2 Tbls. catsup
1/8 Tsp. dried oregano, crushed
1 ea. French roll, split
1 ea slice of fat-free mozzarella
cheese

Crumble the Italian sausage into a
casserole dish. Stir in the chopped
onion. Cook uncovered until
sausage is done, stirring only once.
Drain off the fat. Stir in the catsup
and oregano. Heat the sausage
mixture thoroughly. Place the roll
bottom on tin foil. Spoon the
sausage mixture on top of the roll
bottom, top with a slice of cheese
and cover with the roll top. Wrap
up in the foil and put in oven for
ten minutes or until cheese is
melted.

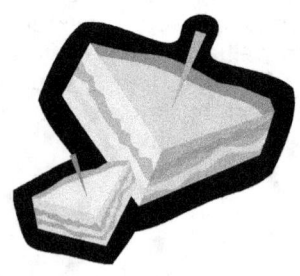

Salads

Herb Salad

Head of Red Lettuce
4 fresh, vine-ripened tomatoes,
sliced
small red onion, diced thinly
¼ c. chopped fresh basil
1/8 c. chopped fresh sage
1/8 c. chopped fresh mint
1/3 c. extra-virgin olive oil
3 tbsp. balsamic vinegar
Salt and pepper to taste

Mix all the ingredients thoroughly.
Serve chilled.

Spinach Salad

small pkg. fresh spinach
1 large mild onion, cut into rings
1 large orange
Orange juice- unsweetened
2 Tsp. Olive oil
1 clove garlic
½ Tsp. salt
¼ Tsp. freshly ground pepper

Wash spinach, remove tough stems and discard; pat leaves dry and tear into pieces. Place in a salad bowl. Add onion rings. Peel orange and remove sections with knife. Cut each section in half; add to spinach. Squeeze juice from remaining orange membrane into a cup; pour in enough additional orange juice to make ¼c. Add oil, garlic, salt and pepper to orange juice; stir well. Pour over spinach mixture; toss to mix well. Cover and refrigerate for 4 hours before serving.

Salad to Go

1 can low-sodium garbanzo beans
1 pint cherry tomatoes, preferably sweet grape variety
1 can sliced ripe olives, drained
4 ounces sliced mushrooms
½ medium green bell pepper, chopped
1c. cooked, diced, skinless, boneless chicken breast
5c. chopped Green leaf lettuce
2/3c. cider vinegar
1 ½ Tbls. extra-virgin olive oil
2 packets sugar substitute

1 Tsp. dried oregano leaves
¼ Tsp. black pepper

Place beans and cherry tomatoes in colander and run under cold water until rinsed. In large mixing bowl, combine bean mixture, olives, mushrooms, bell pepper, and chicken; toss gently to blend. Place equal amounts of salad mixture into 5 gallon-sized plastic re-sealable bags. In measuring cup combine vinegar, olive oil, sugar substitute, oregano, and black pepper. Whisk until well blended. Spooning 3 Tbls. of dressing into 5 small plastic re-sealable bags then seal and place one in each of the salad bags. Seal and refrigerate until needed.

To transport, add 1 c. of lettuce to each salad bag the day the salad is being served. Do not add lettuce prior to that time or it will become limp.

To serve, pour dressing into gallon-size bag with salad. Seal bag and toss to coat salad with dressing.

Pasta Vegetable Salad

2 Tbsp cider vinegar
2 Tbsp tomato sauce
2 tsp sugar substitute
2 Tbsp olive oil
1 garlic clove, minced
¼ tsp basil
salt and pepper to taste
1 c. uncooked penne pasta
1 large tomato, diced
1 small zucchini, diced
1 medium red or yellow pepper,
seeded & chopped
1 c. broccoli
1 c. cauliflower

Combine vinegar and tomato sauce
in a large serving bowl; stir to mix
well. Stir in the sugar, oil, garlic,
basil, salt, and pepper; set to the
side. Cook the pasta according to
package directions. Transfer to a
colander and rinse under cold,
running water; drain. Meanwhile,
add the tomatoes, zucchini,
pepper, cauliflower, and broccoli to
the bowl with the dressing. Stir to
mix well. Stir in the pasta and
serve immediately or cover and
refrigerate up to 36 hours before
serving.

Chicken Salad

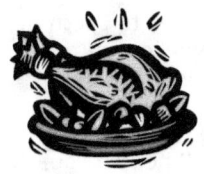

3 c. cooked chicken, diced
1 apple, diced
½ c. sliced green onions
1 c. red grapes (seedless)
1 c. green grapes (seedless)
½ c. chopped celery
1 c. non-fat plain yogurt
1 Tbsp lemon juice
1 tsp dry mustard
1 tsp dried dill weed
Salt & pepper to taste
3 c. cooked wild rice

In a large bowl, combine the chicken, apple, green onions, grapes, and celery. In a small bowl, whisk together the yogurt, lemon juice, mustard, dill, salt, and pepper. Combine the cooked wild rice and chicken mixture. Toss with the dressing and serve.

Grilled Vegetable Salad

2 baby eggplants cut in half
1 medium yellow summer squash,
cut in half lengthwise
1 medium zucchini, cut in half
lengthwise
1 green bell pepper, quartered
1 red bell pepper, quartered
1 small onion, cut in half
½ c. orange juice, unsweetened
2 Tbls. lime juice
1 Tbls. olive oil
2 cloves garlic, minced
1 Tsp. dried oregano leaves
salt to taste
¼ Tsp. ground red pepper
¼ Tsp. black pepper
2 Tbls. chopped fresh cilantro

Combine all ingredients except
cilantro in large bowl; toss to coat.
To prevent sticking, spray grill with
non-stick cooking spray. Prepare
coals for cooking and place
vegetables on grill, 2 to 3 inches
from hot coals; reserve marinade.
Grill until tender and lightly
charred; reserving the marinade.
Broil 2 to 3 inches from heat, 3 to
4 minutes per side or until tender;
cool 10 minutes. Remove peel from
eggplant. Slice vegetables into

bite-size pieces; return to
marinade. Stir in cilantro; toss to
coat.

Chicken Salad (Mom Style)

12 oz. sliced chicken
½ c. chopped celery
¼ c. shredded carrots
¼ c. salad fat-free dressing
1 ½ Tsp. line juice
Salt and pepper to taste

Combine cooked chicken, celery,
and carrots in large bowl and set
aside. Stir the dressing, juice, salt,
and pepper in a small bowl and mix
well. Pour this over the chicken
mixture. Making sure to toss it and
coat it well.

Italian Potato Salad

24 new red potatoes washed
3 stalks celery, chopped
1 red bell pepper, diced
¼ c. chopped green onions
Dressing:
2 Tbsp olive oil
1 Tbsp balsamic vinegar
½ Tbsp red vinegar
1 tsp fresh parsley, chopped
Fresh ground pepper to taste

Boil the potatoes for 20 minutes in a large pot of boiling water. Drain and let cool for 30 minutes. Cut cooled potatoes into large chunks and toss them with the celery, red pepper, and green onions.

Combine the oil, vinegar, parsley, and pepper together and pour over the potato salad. Serve at room temperature.

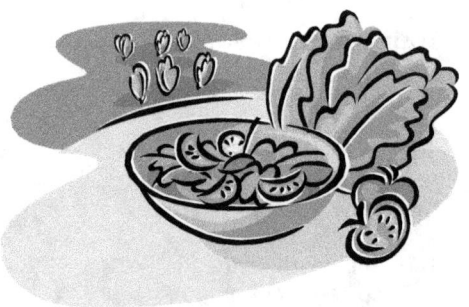

Side Dishes

Stuffed Mushrooms

12 medium mushrooms
½ c. shredded process cheese
¼ c. Seasoned Bread crumbs
1 tsp water

Clean mushrooms and remove
stems, making sure to reserve the
mushroom caps. Chop stems and
measure 1/3 c. lightly melt the
cheese until soft. Blend in bread
crumbs, chopped stems, and
water. Work mixture with hands
into 12 balls. Place one in each
mushroom cap. Place on a baking
sheet with non-stick spray. Bake in
a 400 degree oven for 10 minutes.

Stuffed Cabbage Rolls

1 Cabbage (medium size head)
Filling -
1 lb. Extra Lean Ground Beef
1 c. Cooked Rice
½ Tsp. Garlic Powder
1 Egg or egg substitute

Sauce -
1 ½ c. Tomato Juice
1 Tbsp. Vinegar, White or Cider
2 Tbsp. Sugar Substitute
1/3 c. Tomato Paste

Place head of cabbage in large pot; adding water to cover. Heat over high heat and boil for 15 minutes, or until soft. Remove cabbage from heat; drain and cool completely. Remove hard outer veins from the leaves; set to the side. Preheat oven to 350 degrees. Combine beef, rice, garlic powder, and egg in a large mixing bowl. Stir until well blended. Place a small amount (approx. 1/3c.) of meat mixture into the center of a cabbage leaf. Fold cabbage leaf over, tucking in the sides to keep meat mixture inside the cabbage leaf. Place cabbage rolls in an 8x8 pan. Whisk all remaining ingredients together in a small mixing bowl until smooth. Spoon sauce over the cabbage rolls. Bake in preheated 350 degree oven for 1 hour.

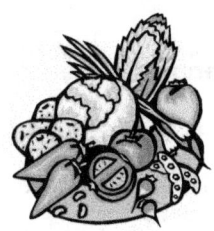

Sweat N' Sour Cabbage

4 c. shredded cabbage
3 oz. ham
2 tbsp. artificial brown sugar or sugar
substitute
2 tbsp. Flour
¼ c. water
1/3 c. vinegar
1 small onion sliced
2 cloves
Salt and pepper to taste

Cook the cabbage in boiling salted
water for 7 minutes. Add your
sugar and flour to small amount of
bouillon; blend to a fine mixture.
Add in the water, vinegar, cloves,
salt, and pepper; stir and cook
until thick. Then add your onion,
ham, and cabbage. Mix up well.
Heat thoroughly and serve warm.

Macaroni and Cheese

2 c. elbow macaroni
½ c. egg substitute
1 Tsp. no-salt seasoning mix
½ Tsp. black pepper
1 c. low-fat cheddar cheese
1 c. low-fat American cheese
3 Tsp. light margarine
½ Tsp. paprika
4 c. skim milk
salt to taste

Bring ½ gallon water to boil, add macaroni noodles, and stir. As soon as the water has come to a rapid boil, cook for another 3-5 minutes until tender. Turn off heat and drain the noodles and immediately rinse with cold water. Drain and set to the side. Combine egg substitute with the milk, then add all seasonings; mix well. Mix all cheeses and margarine with the macaroni. Spray a four-quart casserole dish with non-stick spray. Pour macaroni-cheese mixture in the prepared casserole dish. Pour the egg - milk mixture over the macaroni. Bake at 350 degrees or approximately 30-40 minutes or until bubbly.

Scalloped Potatoes

2 medium potatoes, peeled and
thinly sliced
1 small onion, chopped
2 Tsp. flour
Salt and pepper to taste
1 ½c. skim milk
1 Tsp. light, soft-tub margarine
2 Tbls. Parmesan cheese

Preheat or toaster oven to 350
degrees. Place half the potatoes in
a baking dish. Scatter the onions
over them. Sprinkle with flour, salt,
and pepper. Place remaining
potatoes on top of the onions. Heat
the milk and simmer. Pour the milk
over the potatoes, dot with
margarine, and sprinkle with
cheese. Bake for about 1 hour until
potatoes are tender.

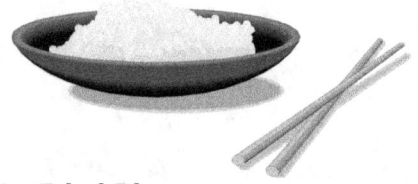

Un-Fried Rice

¾ c. + 1 Tbsp (uncooked) rice
1 ¾ c. chicken stock
1 ½ c. lean ham
¼ c. diced onions
2 Tbsp bias-cut celery
¼ c. + 3 Tbsp diced carrots
¼ c. diced red pepper
¼ c. diced green pepper
½ tsp garlic powder
1/16 tsp ground ginger
1 Tbsp soy sauce
¼ tsp red pepper flakes
½ c. frozen peas, thawed
3/8 tsp margarine
1 small egg substitute
1 Tbsp chopped green onions

Cook the rice in the chicken stock
in a covered saucepan until tender
and firm. Heat the ham, onions,
celery, carrots, red and green
peppers, rice, garlic powder,
ginger, soy sauce, and red pepper
flakes for 20 minutes in a large
saucepan on low heat. Add peas
and mix with rice. Set aside. Melt

margarine in a small skillet. Add beaten egg and scramble until firm. Set aside. Transfer rice mixture to serving platter. Chop up the scramble eggs and sprinkle over rice mixture. Sprinkle chopped green onions over top to garnish.

Pasta Primavera

1 c. noodles, uncooked
1 Tbls. vegetable oil
2 c. chopped mixed vegetables of your choice
1c. chopped tomatoes
¼ Tsp. garlic powder
1/8 Tsp. black pepper
3 Tbls. Parmesan cheese

Cook noodles according to package directions. Now, while noodles are cooking, heat oil in a skillet. Add vegetables and sauté until tender; stir constantly. Add tomato and sauté 2 more minutes. Toss vegetables with noodles. Add seasonings; sprinkle with Parmesan cheese.

Green Bean Casserole

1 package of green beans
1 can condensed low-fat cream of mushroom soup
¼ Tsp. ground black pepper
1 onion, thinly sliced into rings
¼ c. chopped walnuts
2 Tbls. parmesan cheese
1 ½ Tbls. Seasoned bread-crumbs

Preheat oven to 350 degrees. In a large bowl, combine green beans, mushroom soup, and pepper. Toss to mix gently. Coat a 2 quarter casserole dish with cooking spray. Place the green bean mixture into the casserole. Arrange the onion rings on top of the green beans. Sprinkle the casserole with walnuts, cheese, and bread crumbs. Bake for about 40 to 50 minutes until bubbly and lightly browned on top.

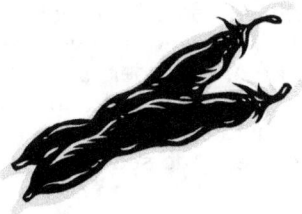

Meats

Spicy Shrimp and Garlic

1 c. Olive Oil
1 Juice from a small lemon
½ Tbls. Paprika
1 ea Bay Leaf
1 Tbls. Crushed Rosemary leaves
¼ Tbls. Cayenne Pepper
1 Dash Tabasco Sauce
1 Dash of salt
1 Dash of pepper
1 Dash of Worcestershire Sauce
30 ea cloves of Garlic, parboiled and peeled
1 ½ lbs. Shrimp

Gently heat the olive oil in a skillet. Add all the remaining ingredients except the shrimp. Cook very gently for 15 minutes. Raise the heat and stir in the shrimp. Toss the shrimp constantly in the oil, until just pink and begin to curl. Cover and marinate in the refrigerator for a day.

Ginger Ribs with Apricot Glaze

1 slab baby back ribs, app. 2 ½ lbs
2 Tbls. low sugar apricot preserves
1 ½ Tsp. spicy brown mustard
1 Tsp. sugar substitute
1 ½ Tsp. soy sauce
low-sodium seasoning salt

Sprinkle both sides of the slab of ribs generously with low-sodium seasoning salts. Curl the slab around and fit it down into your slow cooker. Cover and set the cooker on low. Forget about it for 9 -10 hours. When the time's up, mix together the preserves, mustard, sugar substitute, and soy sauce. Carefully remove the ribs form the slow cooker - they may fall apart on you a bit. Arrange them meaty-side up on a broiler rack. Spread the apricot glaze evenly over the ribs and put them in a broiler set on high for 7-8 minutes.

Baked Dijon Chicken

¼ c. Dijon mustard
¼ c. evaporated fat-free milk
¼ seasoned bread crumbs
¼c. fat-free grated cheese
4 boneless, skinless chicken breasts

Preheat oven to 425 degrees.
Spray a 13x9 inch baking dish with
non-stick cooking spray. Combine
mustard and evaporated milk in a
shallow bowl. Combine bead
crumbs and cheese in separate
shallow bowl. Dip chicken into
mustard mixture, coating on both
sides, then into bread crumb
mixture. Place on prepared dish.
Bake for 30 minutes.

HAM AND SWISS QUICHE
WITH MUSHROOMS

1 c. diced cooked lean ham
1 c. chopped mushrooms
2 green onions sliced
4 eggs or egg substitute
1 ½ c. skim milk
2 tbsp. melted butter
1 tsp Worcestershire sauce
½ c. all purpose flour
½ tsp salt
¼ tsp black pepper

Dash cayenne

Preheat oven to 350 degrees. Lightly spray a deep pie pan with non-stick cooking spray. Sprinkle the cheese, ham, mushrooms, and green onion in layers. In a deep bowl, beat together eggs, milk, butter, Worcestershire, flour, salt, pepper, and cayenne. Pour over ingredients in pie pan. Bake for 40 to 50 minutes, or until a knife inserted in the center comes out clean. Cool for 5 to 10 minutes. Serve.

Red Snapper Fillet

¼ c. low-sodium chicken broth
¼ c. lemon juice
½ Tsp. dried oregano
½ Tsp. dried basil
¼ Tsp. salt
¼ Tsp. pepper
4 cloves garlic, minced
1 can salt-free diced tomatoes, drained

Place fish in a baking dish. Combine broth, lemon juice, oregano, basil, salt, pepper, and garlic; make sure to stir well. Pour broth mixture and tomatoes over fish. Cook immediately, uncovered, at 350 degrees for 25 minutes or until fish flakes easily when tested with a fork.

Baked Pork Chops in Sour-Cream Gravy

6 ea Pork Chops
1 ea Garlic Clove, minced
1 Tsp. Caraway Seed, crushed
2 Tsp. Paprika, mild
1 Dash of Salt
1 Dash of pepper
1 c. White Wine, Dry
1 c. Sour Cream (Fat-Free)

Place the pork chops in a casserole dish. Mix the remaining ingredients, except for the sour cream and pour over the chops. Marinate the chops for 2 to 3 hours in the refrigerator. Bake the chops, uncovered in preheated 325 degree oven until tender. Add more wine if necessary. Stir sour cream into pan juices and heat through but do not boil. Serve chops with sour-cream gravy and noodles or dumplings.

RUSTIC CAJUN CHICKEN AND SAUSAGE RICE

6 oz. pork sausage
16 oz. frozen mixed pepper stir-fry, thawed
½ c. chopped onion
¾ c. sliced celery
½ Tsp. dried thyme leaves
1 c. water
2 bay leaves
½ c. uncooked white rice
½ Tsp. paprika
8 ounces boneless skinless chicken breast meat, cut into bite-sized pieces
Hot pepper sauce to taste

Place a 12-inch non-stick skillet over medium high heat until hot. Add sausage and cook until no longer pink, breaking up larger pieces while stirring. Remove from skillet and set aside. Add pepper stir-fry, onion, celery, and thyme to pan residue and cook 3-4 minutes; stirring frequently. Increase heat to high, add water and bay leaves, stir and bring to a boil. Add rice and paprika and return to a boil. Reduce heat, cover tightly, and simmer 15 minutes.

Add chicken and cook 5 more minutes or until chicken is no longer pink in center. Remove skillet from heat and stir in sausage and hot pepper sauce. Cover and let stand 5 minutes to absorb flavors.

TERIYAKI PORK CHOPS

6 pork loin chops

Marinade ingredients:
¼ c. light soy sauce
¼ c. dry sherry
2 Tbls. sugar
3 garlic cloves, minced
1 Tbls. peanut oil

Combine all marinade ingredients. Add the pork chops and marinate in the refrigerator for 4-24 hours. Grill or broil the pork chops, turning once, for 12-13 minutes until juices run clear.

Salmon Snow Peas

2 small leeks, white and pale part chopped fine
2 large carrots
½ lb. snow peas

4 salmon steaks or fillets
2 Tsp. grated fresh ginger
2 Tbsp. rice vinegar
1 Tsp. plus 1 Tbsp. sesame oil, divided
Salt and freshly ground black pepper
1 lb. fresh spinach
1 Tbsp. fresh lemon juice

Preheat oven to 450 degrees. Tear four large sheets of heavy-duty aluminum foil and lay out on table or counter. Place one-fourth each of leeks, carrots, and snow peas on each sheet of foil. Place a piece of salmon on top of each mound of vegetables. Sprinkle one-fourth of the ginger and drizzle one-fourth of the vinegar and one-fourth Tsp. oil over each piece of fish; season to taste with salt and pepper. Double-fold foils and seals tightly, to form four packets. (Leave enough room in the packet for heat to circulate.) Place packets on cookie sheet and bake about 20 minutes, or until fish flakes easily with fork. Meanwhile, rinse spinach leaves and place in large bowl or platter that will fit in a microwave oven. Drizzle with fresh lemon juice and remaining 1 Tbls.. oil. Cook in microwave at high power 3-4 minutes, checking every minute or so to make sure spinach is tender but not over-cooked. Place one-fourth of spinach in center of each of 4 plates, making a flat bed. While opening the packets, be careful to allow steam to escape the opening first without scalding your hands. Transfer contents to the top of the bed of spinach on each plate.

GRILLED PEPPER PORK

6 pork loin chops, about 1 inch thick
Marinate Ingredients:
2 garlic cloves, crushed
1 Tbls. crushed coriander seeds
8 crushed black pepper or white peppercorns
1 Tsp. brown sugar
3 Tbls. light soy sauce

Combine all ingredients except the pork chops, then add the chops and marinate for 30 minutes. Grill or broil the chops, brushing with marinade and turning once, for about 12-14 minutes.

Sweet N' Sour Pork

¼ lb. lean boneless pork
2 Tsp. canola Oil
1 Tsp. sesame oil
1 ea small carrot
½ small green bell pepper, sliced into strips
1 green onion, sliced
2 Tbls. brown sugar or substitute
1 Tsp. cornstarch
1 Tbls. water
1 Tbls. red wine vinegar
½ Tsp. soy sauce
1 dash ginger
½c. pineapple chunks, drained
side order of hot cooked rice

Partially freeze pork and slice, thinly, into strips. Preheat a non-stick frying pan. Add the Canola and Sesame oil to pan; swirl to coat the dish. Add the pork and cook covered until pork is no longer pink, turning every 30 seconds. Stir in sliced carrot, green pepper, and sliced green onion. Cook covered until the vegetables are crisp and tender. Drain off remaining liquid. In a small bowl mix together the brown sugar and cornstarch then stir in the water, vinegar, soy sauce, and ground ginger. Cook uncovered until thickened and bubbles. Stir in drained pineapple chunks. Cook again, uncovered until the pineapple is heated thoroughly. Toss the pineapple mixture with the pork mixture and serve with the side of hot cooked rice.

Chicken with Sausage in Tomato Sauce

¼ c. olive oil
4 ea large cloves garlic
2 ½ lbs. sausage links
1 ½ lbs. hot sausage links
4 ea chicken legs
4 ea chicken thighs
2 cans tomatoes, diced
1 can tomato paste
1 dash of salt and pepper

Heat oil in a large skillet; add the garlic and sauté until lightly golden. Remove the garlic and set aside. Prick the sausages in several places and sear them in the hot oil. Remove and set them aside, covered. Brown the chicken on all sides in the same skillet. Remove and cover it. Pour 1 tbs of the drippings into a large casserole dish. Discard the remaining drippings. Pour the tomatoes in with the drippings and add the tomato paste, salt, pepper, basil, and the garlic. Simmer for 15 minutes uncovered. Add the sausage and simmer for 20 minutes, covered. Add the chicken, cover and simmer for 20 more minutes.

Broccoli, Chicken and Rice Casserole

2 c. white rice
2 c. boiling water
4 boneless, skinless chicken breasts
¼ Tsp. garlic powder
2 c. frozen broccoli
1 c. reduced-fat shredded Cheddar cheese

Heat oven to 425°F. In 13×9-inch baking pan, combine the rice, salt, and pepper to taste. Add boiling water; mix well. Add chicken; sprinkle with garlic powder. Cover and bake 30 minutes. Add broccoli and cheese; continue to bake, covered, 8 to 10 minutes or until chicken is no longer pink in center.

Baked Ranch Parmesan Chicken

6 chicken breasts halves
½ c. light ranch dressing
1 c. seasoned bread crumbs
½ c. low-fat Parmesan cheese
1 Tsp. cracked black pepper
1 Tsp. sage
½ Tsp. salt

Marinate chicken in the ranch dressing for 4 hours or overnight. Preheat oven to 450*F. Combine bread crumbs, Parmesan cheese, black pepper, sage, and salt; mix well. Coat the marinated breasts in breading mixture and place in a baking dish. Bake for 20 minutes, then reduce to 350*F and bake for additional 30 minutes or until done and juices run clear.

Canadian Style Pizza

Thin-crust bread shell
1 c. Pizza Sauce
2/3 c. skim milk
6 oz. low-fat mozzarella cheese
Canadian bacon, cut into bite-size pieces
1 small onion, cut into thin rings
½ c. thinly sliced fresh mushrooms

1 small green bell pepper, cut into thin rings
½ Tsp. crushed dried oregano
½ Tsp. crushed dried basil
crushed red pepper flakes (optional)

Preheat oven to 450 degree. Place the shell on an un-greased non-stick pizza pan. To assemble the pizza, spread the pizza sauce over the shell, leaving a 1-inch border around the rim. Sprinkle with half of the cheese. Arrange the Canadian bacon on top of the cheese; covering evenly. Top with mushroom slices, onions, and bell pepper rings. Sprinkle evenly with oregano, basil, and red pepper flakes (if using). Top with remaining cheese. Bake for 13 to 15 minutes, until the crust is crisp and the cheese is melted and browned.

CHICKEN FINGERS

3 boneless, skinless breast halves, sliced into long strips
2 egg whites or egg substitute, fork beaten
¾ tsp garlic powder
¾ tsp onion powder

¾ tsp seasoning salt
¾ tsp parsley flakes
1 tbsp cornflake crumbs

Coat chicken strips with egg whites in medium bowl. Stirring until chicken is coated. Combine the garlic powder, onion powder, seasoning salt, parsley, and cornflake crumbs in a large bowl. Dip chicken strips in and coat evenly; place on lightly greased baking sheet. Lightly spray surfaces of coated chicken strips with cooking spray for crispness. Bake on 400 degrees for 10 minutes. Turn strips over and bake for 10 more minutes, until chicken is no longer pink.

Garlic Meat Loaf

1 c. quick cooking oats
½ c. fat-free milk
2 egg whites or egg substitute
¼ c. catsup
½ c. chopped onion
¼ c. chopped green bell pepper
1 clove garlic, minced
1 Tsp. seasoning
1-1/2 pounds lean ground beef
¾ Tsp. salt

½ Tsp. pepper

Mix oats, milk, egg whites, catsup, onion, bell pepper, garlic, and herbs in medium bowl. Mix in beef, salt, and pepper until blended. Pat mixture into un-greased loaf pan or shape into a loaf in baking pan. Bake at 350 degrees until juices run clear about 1 hour. Let stand in pan for 5 minutes before serving.

Turkey Hash

¼ c. chopped onion
2 Tbls. chicken stock
1 c. diced skinless cooked turkey
1 can low-fat cream of celery soup
1 ½ c. cooked diced potato
2/3 c. cooked green peas
¼ c. shredded fat-free American cheese
Paprika

Preheat oven to 350 degrees. Sauté onion in chicken stock in non-stick skillet until tender. Add turkey, soup, potatoes, and peas. Place mixture in 1-quart non-stick casserole. Top with shredded cheese and paprika. Bake for 30 minutes.

PORK CUTLETS WITH BACON

2 slices lean bacon
1 large onion, cut in half and sliced
2 Tsp. balsamic vinegar
Non-stick cooking spray
4 pork cutlets, trimmed of excess fat
½ Tsp. salt
¼ Tsp. fresh ground black pepper

Cook the bacon in a large non-stick skillet for about 6 minutes. Remove the bacon from the skillet and chop it into bite-sized pieces. Drain all but 1 Tsp. of the fat. Add the onion to the skillet and cook for 7-8 minutes. Add the balsamic vinegar and cook for 1 minute. Remove the onions from the skillet. Add the bacon to the onions and keep warm. Wipe the skillet clean and spray with cooking spray. Sprinkle the pork with salt and pepper and sauté the pork over medium heat for 4-5 minutes per side. Serve the bacon and onion mixture over the pork.

Deserts

Frozen Banana Yogurt

1 c. low-fat banana-cream pudding
1 c. flavored low-fat yogurt
1 c. mashed banana
1 tsp. vanilla extract
½ tsp. banana extract

Combine all the ingredients in a
food processor. Pour into two small
yogurt containers; freeze for a few
hours or overnight.

Easy chocolate Graham Torte

2 pkg. sugar-free chocolate pudding
1 box of graham crackers

Line a 9 X 13 pan with a layer of
graham crackers. Prepare 1
package of pudding as directed on
the package. Spread over the
graham cracker layer. Put down
another layer of graham crackers
squares over the pudding. Prepare

second package of pudding and
spread over the top of that layer of
graham crackers. Cover the bowl
and refrigerate. When ready to
serve torte, spread top with
whipped cream.

Lemon Cheesecake

Crust:
4 full graham cracker sheets
¼ c. melted butter

Filling Ingredients:
1 4 oz. pkg. un-sweetened lemon
Jello
1 c. boiling water
1 -8 oz. package low-fat cream
cheese
¼ c. sugar substitute
1 Tsp. lemon juice
1 8 oz light Cool whip

 To make the crust:
Crush the graham crackers into
fine crumbs and mix with melted
butter. Press onto the bottom of a
9" pie pan.
Mix the Jello powder with the
boiling water and let stand until it
just begins to gel. Set aside. In a
large bowl, beat the cream cheese,

sugar substitute, and lemon juice until smooth and well blended. Next, add the Jello and beat very, very well. Fold in the cool whip and pour into crust. Chill several hours.

Dreamy Orange Pound Cake

1 white cake mix
2 un-sweetened orange Jello mix
1 8 oz. light cool whip
2 ½ c. warm water

Follow instructions on cake mix and bake. When cake is done, let cool then poke holes all over cake. Set to the side. Mix the Jello by following the box instructions; pour over cake filling up holes. Top with cool whip and chill for 2 hours.

Easy Fudge

¼ c. diet margarine
2 oz. unsweetened chocolate
1 c. sugar substitute
1 Tsp. vanilla extract
1 pkg. light cream cheese

Optional: ½c. chopped nuts

Melt margarine over low heat. Add

chocolate and stir just until melted. Remove from heat and stir in sweetener and vanilla. Combine chocolate mixture with cream cheese and beat until smooth. Stir in the nuts (optional). Spread mixture in a lightly greased 8 inch square pan. Refrigerate until firm.

Grilled Banana Split

1 large ripe firm banana
½ Tsp. melted butter
2 Tbls. fat-free chocolate syrup
2/3 c. sugar-free vanilla ice cream
2 Tbls. toasted sliced almonds

Prepare hot coals on grill for cooking. Cut unpeeled bananas lengthwise; brush melted butter over cut sides. Grill bananas, cut side down, over medium-hot coals 2 minutes or until lightly browned; turn and grill 2 minutes or until tender. Cut bananas in half crosswise; be careful to remove the peel gently. Place 2 pieces of banana in each bowl;
top with 1/3 c. ice cream
1 Tbls. chocolate syrup
1 Tbls. almonds; serve immediately.

Sweetheart Shortcakes

3 c. fresh sliced berries mixed
2 Tbls. finely chopped crystallized ginger
1-2/3 c. all-purpose flour
1 Tbls. sugar substitute
2 Tsp. baking powder
¼ Tsp. baking soda
3 Tbls. light margarine
½ c. buttermilk
¼ c. egg substitute
Non-stick cooking spray
1 4 oz light cool whip
¼ c. fat-free dairy sour cream

In a small bowl combine the berries and the crystallized ginger. Set aside. Meanwhile, prepare shortcakes.

For shortcakes; in a medium bowl stir together flour, sugar, baking powder, and baking soda. Using a pastry blender, cut in butter or margarine until the mixture resembles coarse crumbs. Combine buttermilk and egg substitute. Add to the flour mixture all at once, stirring just until mixture is moistened. Lightly coat a baking sheet with cooking spray and set to the side. On a lightly floured surface pat the dough to ½ -inch thickness. Cut the dough with a floured 2 ½ -inch heart-shaped or star-shaped cookie cutter or a round biscuit cutter, re-rolling scraps as necessary. Place shortcakes on prepared baking sheet. Bake in a 425 degree oven until golden brown. Cool the shortcakes slightly on a wire rack. To serve, in a small bowl combine the whipped topping and sour cream. Split shortcakes in half. Place bottoms on dessert plates. Divide the berry mixture among bottoms. Top each with some of the whipped topping mixture. Replace the shortcake tops.

Sugar-Free Chocolate Pie

Crust:
4 sheets of graham crackers
¼ c. of melted butter

Filling:
1 small package sugar-free chocolate pudding
1 small package sugar-free butterscotch pudding
¼ Tsp. almond extract or flavoring

2 ½ c. skim milk
1 8 oz. tub of Light Cool Whip

Prepare crust and side to the side.
Mix chocolate and butterscotch
puddings with the milk. Pour into
crust. Add ¼ Tsp. almond flavoring
to Cool Whip and mix. Cover top of
pie completely with Cool Whip
mixture. Refrigerate before
serving.

Sugar Free Peach Popovers

1 can sugar-free cling peaches,
drained,
2 Tsp. cinnamon
1 envelope artificial sweetener
½ Tsp. salt
1 Tsp. cornstarch
½ c. raisins
1 package crescent rolls

Combine the peaches, cinnamon,
sweetener, salt, cornstarch and
raisins together. Open the crescent
rolls and pat them out flat. Put
several spoonfuls of filling into the
center of each roll. Fold over pastry
dough to form triangle. Bake on
un-greased cookie sheet at 375
degrees approximately 45 minutes.

For glazed top, baste lightly with egg white before cooking.

Pumpkin Pie

Crust:
4 sheets graham crackers
¼ c. of butter

Filling:
can Pumpkin Puree
¾ c. sugar substitute
2 Tbsp. Corn Starch
½ Tsp. Cinnamon
1 ½ Tsp. Pumpkin Pie Spice
1/8 Tsp. Salt
½ c. Fat Free Half-and-Half
½ c. Egg Substitute
3 Tbsp. Heavy Cream
1 Tbsp. Vanilla

Preheat oven to 400° F. Blend pumpkin puree, sugar substitute, cornstarch, spices, and salt in a medium bowl. Mix until all ingredients are well blended. Add remaining ingredients and mix well. Pour into prepared piecrust. Bake in preheated 400° F oven for 35-40 minutes or until set in the center and the crust is golden brown.

Quick Banana cream Pie

1 Graham Cracker Crust
1 pkg. sugar free vanilla pudding mix
2 bananas firm, ripe

Prepare the sugar free pudding mix. Slice 1 ½ banana into the bottom of Graham crust. Pour pudding over the top. Slice remaining banana and arrange in circle over top. Chill for 2-3 hours.

Beverages

Iced Cappuccino

1 c. fat-free vanilla frozen yogurt or
fat-free vanilla ice cream
1 c. cold strong-brewed coffee
1 Tsp. unsweetened cocoa powder
1 Tsp. vanilla
1 packet sugar substitute

Place all ingredients in food
processor or blender; process until
smooth. Place container in freezer;
freeze 1 to 2 hours or until top and
sides of mixture are partially
frozen. Scrape sides of container;
process until smooth and frothy.
Garnish as desired. Serve
immediately.

Iced Mocha Cappuccino:
Increase amount of unsweetened
cocoa powder to 1 Tbls... Proceed
as above.

Ice Mint Tea

4 tea bags
10 sprigs fresh mint
5 c. boiling water
½ to 1 c. sugar substitute
3 c. boiling water
2/3 c. fresh lemon juice
1/3 c. fresh orange juice

Put in the tea bags, the mint, and 5 c. boiling water in a large, covered container. Let sit for 30 minutes and steep. Mix sugar and 3 c. boiling water in a smaller container and stir until sugar is dissolved. Add lemon and orange juices. Remove tea bags and add sugar and juice mixture to tea mixture. Stir to combine. Refrigerate until ready to drink. Strain and serve over ice.

Cranberry Grapefruit Cooler

3 c. unsweetened pink-grapefruit juice
2 ½ c. low-calorie cranberry-juice cocktail
2 T. sugar substitute
3 c. cracked ice
6 thin slices of lime

Combine pink-grapefruit juice, cranberry juice, and sweetener of your choice in a large pitcher. Stir to dissolve sweetener. Divide the cracked ice equally among six glasses. Pour juice mixture into glasses. Garnish each glass with a slice of lime.

Virgin Pina Colada

1 c. frozen fat-free non-dairy whipped topping
2 Tbls. crushed pineapple in juice, drained
1 tsp. rum extract
1 tsp. coconut extract
1 c. crushed ice

Place all the ingredients in a food processor or blender; process at the highest speed until the ice is liquefied.

Merry Cherry Punch

1 can cherry juice blend
2 Tbsp sugar substitute
Juice and peel of 1 lemon
½ tsp whole cloves
1 cinnamon stick
1 lemon, thinly sliced (for garnish)

Combine all ingredients in large saucepan. Simmer over low heat 10 minutes or until hot. Remove and discard lemon peel, cloves, and cinnamon stick. Carefully pour into heat-proof punch bowl. Garnish with lemon slice.

Digestive Problems Associated with Diabetes

It is estimated that over half of all people with diabetes will have some sort of problem with their digestive tract (also know as the gastrointestinal tract). Although no one really knows the reasons for all of these digestive problems, it seems to be linked to a person's blood sugar and its control, cigarette smoking, and a lower level of "good" cholesterol, also known as HDL (high-density lipo protein).

People with diabetes should be aware of the signs and symptoms of digestive problems. You should also know how to manage these different digestive problems, just incase they develop in the near future.

Warning Signs and Treatment

The most common signs of digestive diabetes are nausea and vomiting. Other symptoms include heart burn, constantly feeling full, getting full easily once you start to eat, slight abdominal pain and abdominal bloating. You may also have symptoms that note the presence of impotence, abnormal sweating, and or dizziness. People with mild to moderate problems may find that it takes longer for food to leave their stomach, while the liquids will leave them normally. Treatment includes changing your diet and tightening up on the control of your blood sugar. Changes to your diet may include cutting back on the intake of high fiber foods, fats, and or increasing the number of feedings from three to six or more smaller meals a day.

Other Digestive Problems

Other common complaints of gastro-paresis include constipation and diarrhea. Diarrhea is recognized by episodes of multiple loose stools, which often occur at night. People with this problem should follow a meal plan designed to meet their nutrient needs, have adequate fluid intake, supplement their diet with a multivitamin, and for those who have diarrhea constantly may even need to take an anti-diarrhea medication. Although diarrhea can be a problem, constipation is the biggest, most common digestive problem that people will have. Doctors consider constipation to be less than three bowel movements per week and it appears to be more common in inactive people. Medications can also cause constipation, such as: antacids. It is extremely important to be sure of what and when you eat. If your digestive system is disrupted, control becomes very difficult. Treatment should include an assessment and discontinuation of unnecessary medications, a diet high in fiber, adequate liquids, tight control of your blood sugar, and regular activity. Treatment should also be started as soon as possible when digestive problems arise. If constipation persists, talk to your diabetes educator or physician. Remember, however, that introducing new medications or discontinuing old ones should be carefully monitored by your diabetes management team.

INFECTIONS

Infections commonly come along
with diabetes and can be very
dangerous. Your blood sugar levels
can rise unexpectedly and be hard
to control when you have an
infection. Common infections
include: ear, mouth, sinus, urinary
tract and skin diseases.

Ear Infections

Symptoms include severe
headaches, a loss of hearing,
fever, and chills. If any of these
symptoms persist you will need to
contact a physician immediately.
Antibiotics will be needed to aid in
the healing process.

Mouth Infections

Tenderness and swelling of your
gums could be an indication to the
beginning of a mouth infection.
Now everyone knows that gum
disease is not life threatening, but
seek treatment from a dentist,
before the infection gets worse and
you begin to lose your teeth.

Sinus Infections

Sinus infections can spread rapidly.
The symptoms include pain in your
face, persistent headaches, and a
yellowish-white nasal discharge.
Antibiotics may be needed, so
contact your physician if any of
these symptoms appear.

Urinary Tract Infections

People can have a urinary tract
infection and have no symptoms at
all, while others will have a burning
and painful sensation while
urinating. Other symptoms include:
fever, back pain, nausea, and
vomiting. If you experience any of
these symptoms, contact your
physician immediately. It may be
necessary to begin taking
antibiotics.

Skin Diseases in Diabetics

Some problems of these skin
diseases can affect anyone, but

people who have diabetes will get them more easily.

These diseases can include: bacterial infections, fungal infections, and itching.

Bacterial Infections

Bacterial infections can cause styes in your eyes, boils, and can even cause infections around the nails.

Fungal Infections

Fungal infections can create itchy rashes of moist, red areas surrounded by tiny blisters and scales. Common fungal infections include jock itch, athlete's foot, ringworm, and vaginal infection that cause itching.

Itching Infections

Itching infections can be caused by a yeast infection, dry skin, or poor circulation. When poor circulation is the cause of itching, the itchiest areas may be the lower parts of the legs. You may be able to treat itching yourself. Limit how often you bathe, particularly when the humidity is low. Use mild soap with moisturizer and apply skin cream after bathing. Make sure you see your physician if any of these symptoms appear.

Traveling with diabetes supplies

Traveling with diabetes can be a tedious job just trying to keep all of your supplies together. But have no fear; we have a few suggestions to keep you stress free and safe while traveling. If you are flying, remember to notify the airport screener that you have diabetes and are carrying your supplies with you.

The following diabetes-related supplies and equipment are allowed through the checkpoint once they have been screened:

Insulin and dispensing products that are clearly identified and labeled
You can have an unlimited number of unused syringes, but only when accompanied by insulin or other inject-able medication
Lancets, blood glucose meters, blood glucose meter test strips, alcohol swabs, meter-testing solutions
Insulin pump and insulin pump supplies

Glucagons emergency kit clearly identified and labeled
You can also have an unlimited number of used syringes when transported in Sharps disposal container or other similar hard-surface container

Medical Record

If you're traveling, it's a good idea to bring your own "Traveling Medical Record" with you. Many people have their medical records scattered in different places; such as: your general medical records can be in this box or file, while your diabetes records will be in another box or file, and your hospital reports will be somewhere else. Since you never can predict which of these records might be important to help you with your care during a trip? It'd be wise to keep a consolidated condensed version of all this information with you when traveling. Keep it in a carry-on bag, not in a suitcase that will get separated from you.

**Here are some other travel
hints that aren't frequently
mentioned:**

Take spare prescriptions for all
your pills.
Take diabetes-related medications
that you might need, even if you
don't usually use them.
Find out who is a diabetes doctor in
the town that you will be visiting.
You can call the nearest hospital,
and ask the diabetes nurse to
recommend one.

Cute Little Home Remedies for the Family

- If you are choking on an ice cube, don't panic. Simply pour a cup of boiling water down your throat and presto, the blockage will be instantly removed.

- Clumsy? Avoid cutting yourself while slicing vegetables by getting someone else to hold them while you chop away.

- Avoid arguments with the Mrs. about lifting the toilet seat by simply using the sink.

- For high blood pressure sufferers: simply cut yourself and bleed for a few minutes; thus reducing the pressure in your veins.

- A mouse trap, placed on top of your alarm clock, will prevent you from rolling over and going back to sleep after you hit the snooze button.

- If you have a bad cough, take a large dose of laxatives, then you will be afraid to cough. Problem solved.

- Have a bad toothache? Smash your thumb with a hammer and you will forget about the toothache.

Sometimes, we just need to remember what the rules of life really are!!
In a redneck world, there are only two tools that you will need.

- WD-40
- Duct Tape

If it doesn't move and should, use the WD-40 and if it shouldn't move and does, then use the duct tape.

Last but not least, we have a beautiful recipe for all chicken lovers that are just not sure how to tell when poultry is thoroughly cooked.

Baked Stuffed Chicken

6 lb. Chicken
1 c. melted butter
1 c. stuffing
1 c. uncooked popcorn
Salt and pepper to taste

Preheat oven to 350 degrees. Brush chicken well with melted butter, salt, and pepper. Fill cavity with stuffing and popcorn. Place in baking pan with the neck end toward the back of the oven. Listen for the popping sounds. When the chicken's butt blows the oven door open and the chicken flies across the room, you know it's done.

And just imagine, you thought I couldn't cook!

OUR DAILY BREAD........ SERVING THE CATAWBA VALLEY AND SURROUNDING AREAS

Our Daily Bread was founded in November 2005 by Jim and Liqiu Taylor. The Taylor's began Our Daily Bread basically because of the numerous stories they are hearing about various local agencies. These agencies require people who need help to meet various guidelines and requirements. Jim says, "To us, that seems not only selfish, but also ludicrous. I mean, Hello!! What is wrong with this picture here? If you all of a sudden fell down on your luck, lost your job and are about to lose your home because you need the money you have to feed your kids, do you really think that you would have the time and much less the money to drive all over town to the various agencies (especially with the way the extreme gas prices are rising) and then you would have to spend virtually the entire day just to get called for your interview and even that's not a guarantee that you will qualify for their help."

Everyday thousands of Americans go hungry due to various reasons and situations. But while Jim was in China, he noticed that with the millions of people that he saw throughout the city, he hardly ever saw anyone begging on the street. When he asked his wife how could this be? She replied, "The Chinese people are very proud individuals and to them it is (all) their duty to look after their neighbors and if someone is spotted as needing food or clothing there will be someone close by to pick them up to get whatever it is that they need." So after returning to the States the couple decided to try and do their part in hopes of not only setting an example in their community but to also make a difference in someone else's life.

Since November of 2005 they have donated over 4 tons of food, 5 tons of clothing, 1 ton of bedding including a tractor trailer load of mattresses and box springs and around 1 ton of small appliances to the Catawba Valley Community. Jim mentions, "Since we began we have had well over 4,000 people come by and received or they have called us. We have delivered various items that are needed to these people when gas donations are possible. Can you imagine just how much more we could do and help if we had the entire communities support? But because of the lack of support there has been many times that we have had to sadly turn folks away simply because we do not have it here to give."

I asked Mr. Taylor, "What group of people are you helping?" and his reply was very fair. They don't think of people as a group because it tends to lead to stereo-types which is unfair. But they do however extend their hands out first to those who are: Single parents, Elderly, Battered Men and Women, Runaway and abused Children, The Handicap and then of course those who are just on a very limited budget. But no matter who they are, Our Daily Bread well strive hard to keep the thoughts of how the good Lord would handle these things. As he once said, "Hungry? Come, sit at my table and I will feed you. Naked? Come and I will clothe you. Weary? Come and rest with me a while." By keepings these things in mind we feel that if we just follow those examples, we can't go wrong.

The services that Our Daily Bread provides all depends on the funds in hand as well as how much we are able to take in and store for the needy. As in the past and hopefully in the future we will be able to give out: Baked Goods, (Breads, Cakes, Snacks, etc) Canned Goods, Non-Perishables, Clothing, Appliances, Bedding, Gas Cards and with the help of our neighbors, Automobiles. Everything we get and donate is 100% free. If it is donated to us then we will pass it on to those in need and not ask a single penny for it. Our Daily Bread is not (yet) a non-profit organization or a true charity, since they have never applied for charity status. Jim's quote on this is, "The cost of just filing the forms to be a charity cost well over $600.00 and that's way beyond our means at this point, but after learning about the Good Samaritan Act of 1996, it allows us to be able to donate various items as long as those who are accepting these items understands that they were donated to us and in turn we are donating it to them "WITHOUT CHARGE"." They go to great lengths to make sure that every donated food item is not damaged, spoiled or have never been tampered with. All clothing is carefully inspected to make sure it is free from harmful chemicals, stains, rips or tares and then they wash, dry and fold each one before letting them go back out the door. When it comes to appliances they make sure that the person who is receiving them understands that its condition is not known and that it is "AS IS". The Gas cards are purchased by whatever funds the community has decided to donate to them and then those cards are given out to those in need.

As times are hard for everyone we must remember that if we all give back to the community, our landfills would be less busy. Upon asking Jim about donating or volunteering, he said, "Anyone can donate to Our Daily Bread. Individuals, Churches, local

Companies, it doesn't matter because it is about ALL OF US doing OUR part to help out OUR fellow neighbors." All donations will be accepted as long as it is in good shape. Unopened food items, canned goods, clothing, pampers, linens, building supplies that are still in good and reusable conditions (which will go to Habitat for Humanity), operational appliances, tools and computers. You name it, if it can go to someone to help better themselves then they will take it, inspect it, and then donate it back out to the community.

Our Daily Bread's motto is based on a very old Chinese culture where, if you have extra give it freely. If you know of a resource to fill your neighbors need then utilize it and assist your neighbor so that they too may have a happy life.